The Amazing Plant-Based Smoothies Collection

Easy and Tasty Plant-Based Smoothies Recipes to Enjoy Your Diet and Boost Your Day

Dave Ingram

Table of contents

Chocolate Green Smoothie

Preparation time: 5 minutes

Cook time: 0 minutes

Serves 2

Ingredients:

6 ounces (170 g) greens (kale, collards, or spinach) 2 very ripe frozen bananas, halved

3 cups plant-based milk

1 tablespoons cocoa powder 1 teaspoon vanilla extract

Directions:

1.   In a blender, combine the greens, bananas, milk, cocoa powder, and vanilla. Blend until smooth and creamy, then serve.

Nutrition Per Serving:

calories: 225 | fat: 6g | carbs: 42g | protein: 6g | fiber: 8g

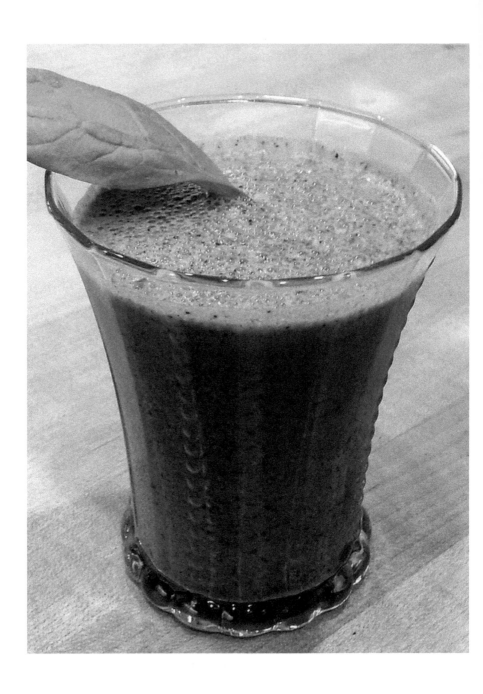

Mango and Pineapple Smoothie

Preparation time: 5 minutes

Cook time: 0 minutes

Serves 2

Ingredients:

2 cups plant-based milk 1 frozen banana

½ cup frozen mango chunks

½ cup frozen pineapple chunks 1 teaspoon vanilla extract

Directions:

1.   In a blender, combine the milk, banana, mango, pineapple, and vanilla. Blend until smooth and creamy, then serve.

Nutrition Per Serving:

calories: 176 | fat: 4g | carbs: 36g | protein: 2g | fiber: 4g

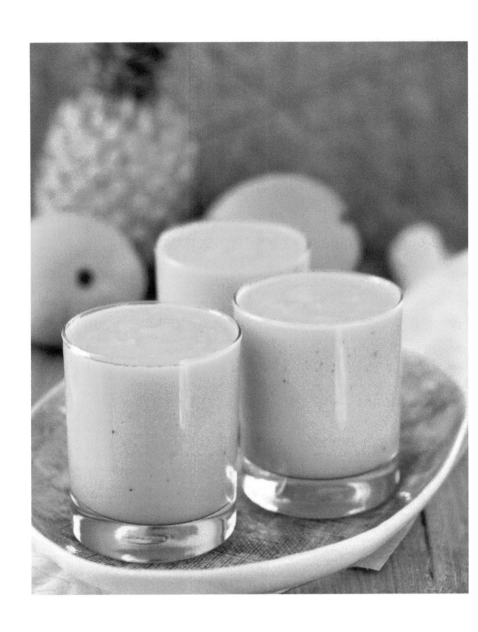

Peanut Butter Banana Smoothie

Preparation time: 5 minutes

Cook time: 0 minutes

Serves 2

Ingredients:

3 frozen bananas, halved 1 cup plant-based milk

2 tablespoons defatted peanut powder 1 teaspoon vanilla extract

½ tablespoon chia seeds

Directions:

1.   Put bananas, milk, peanut powder, and vanilla in a food processor and blend for 2 minutes.

2.   Add the chia seeds, and pulse 2 to 4 times, or until the chia seeds have dispersed evenly without being blended up, and serve.

Nutrition Per Serving:

calories: 271 | fat: 5g | carbs: 47g | protein: 11g | fiber: 8g

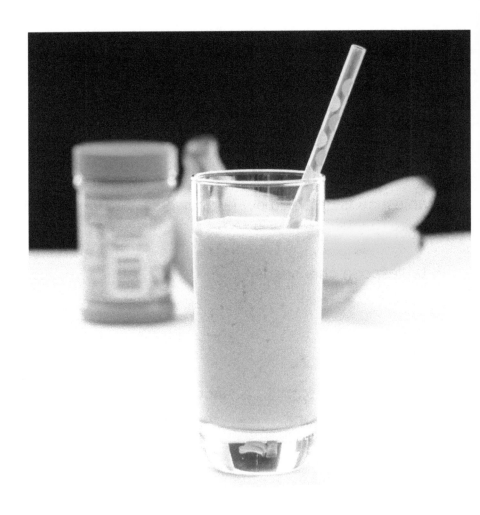

Apple and Walnut Bowl

Preparation time: 15 minutes

Cook time: 0 minutes

Serves 4

Ingredients:

1 green apple, halved, seeded, and cored

3 Honeycrisp apples, halved, seeded, and cored 1 teaspoon freshly squeezed lemon juice

5 pitted Medjool dates

½ teaspoon ground cinnamon Pinch ground nutmeg

2 tablespoons chia seeds, plus more for serving (optional) 1 tablespoon hemp seeds

¼ cup chopped walnuts

Nut butter, for serving (optional)

Directions:

1.   Finely dice half the green apple and 1 Honeycrisp apple.

2.   Coarsely chop the remaining apples and the date

Transfer to a food processor and add the cinnamon a

nutmeg. Pulse to obtain a purée. Stir the purée into t

reserved diced apples. Stir in the chia seeds (if usin

hemp seeds, and walnuts. Refrigerate for at least 1 hc

before serving.

3.   Serve as is or top with additional chia seeds a

nut butter (if using).

Nutrition Per Serving:

calories: 274 | fat: 8g | carbs: 52g | protein: 4g | fib

9g

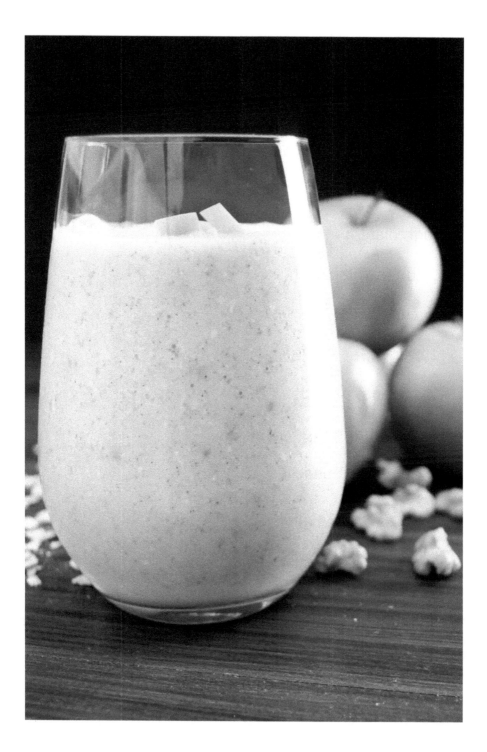

Peach Green Smoothie

Preparation time: 10 minutes

Cook time: 0 minutes

Serves 1

Ingredients:

1 cup fresh spinach

½ cup water

1 orange, peeled

½ banana, peeled

¼ avocado, peeled

½ cup frozen peaches

Directions:

1.   In a high-powered blender, mix the spinach, water, and orange until smooth and juice-like. Add the banana, avocado, and peaches, and mix again.

2.   Serve over ice, if desired.

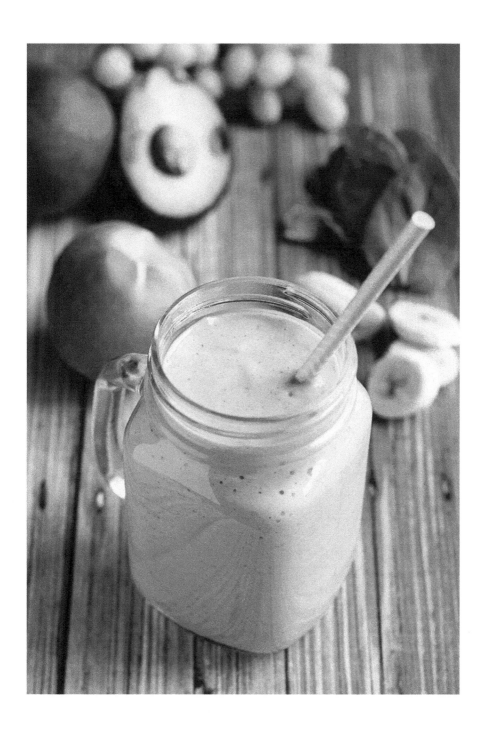

Cake Batter Protein Smoothie

Preparation time: 5 minutes

Cook time: 0 minutes

Serves 2

Ingredients:

1 large banana, frozen

1 cup almond milk (alternatively use soy milk)

¼ cup quick oats

4 tablespoons vegan protein powder (chocolate flavor) 1 tablespoon cashew butter

1 teaspoon cinnamon

1 teaspoon pure vanilla extract

¼ teaspoon nutmeg

Directions:

1.   Mix the oats and almond milk in a small bowl or jar.

2.   Place the bowl in the fridge until the oats have softened, for about 1 hour.

3.   Add the oats and milk mixture along with the remaining ingredients to a blender.

4.   Blend on   high speed   until it   is   smooth   and all   lumps   have disappeared.

5.   Serve in tall glasses with an extra sprinkle of cinnamon on top, or store to enjoy later.

Per Serving

calories: 241 | fat: 7g | carbs: 27g | protein: 16g | fiber: 2g

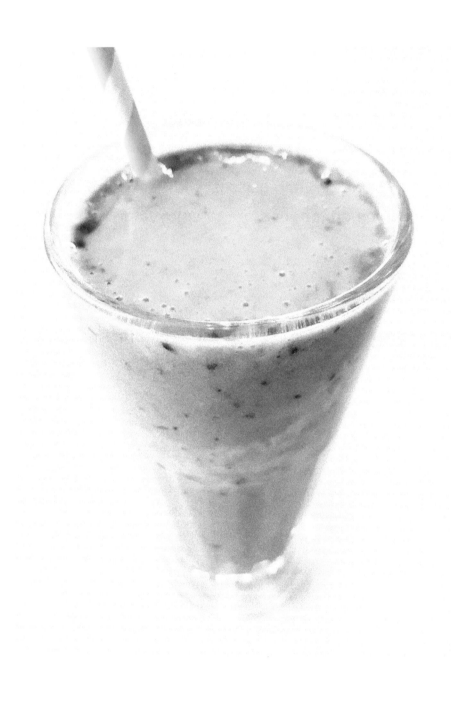

Orange Cardamom Beet Smoothie

Preparation time: 10 minutes

Servings: 1-2

Ingredients:

2 pinches of ground cardamom

1-inch piece of fresh ginger peeled 1 small beet, peeled

1 cup orange juice

1 large frozen banana

Directions:

1.   Put together the ingredients in a food processor.

2.   Blitz until smooth and combined.

3.   Pour into chilled glasses and serve. Enjoy!

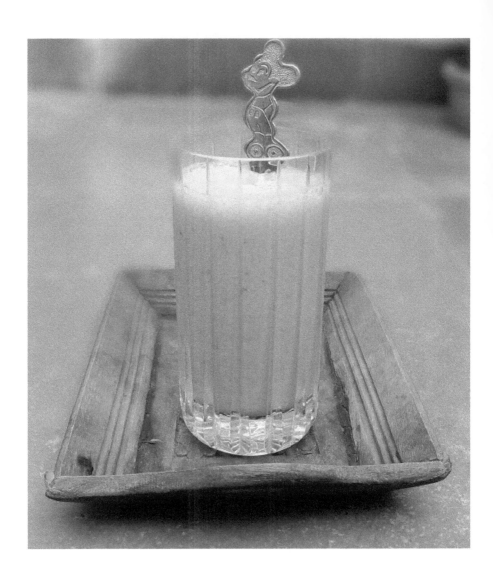

Peachy Mango Smoothie

Preparation time: 5 minutes

Servings: 4

Ingredients:

1 banana

1/4 teaspoon ginger 7 oz peach chunks

2 pinches of turmeric 5 oz mangoes

1 cup of orange juice

Instructions:

1. Put the ingredients in a food processor.

2. Blitz until smooth and combined.

3. Pour into chilled glasses and serve. Enjoy!

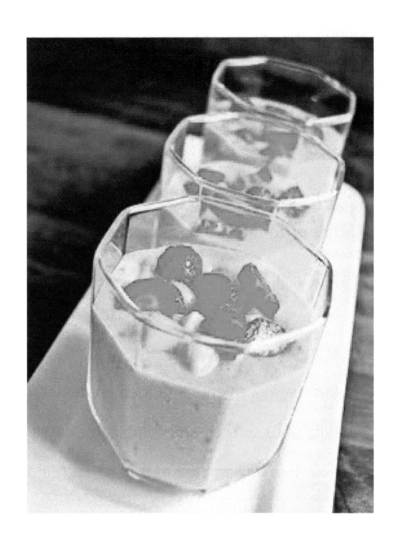

Ginger and Spinach Green Smoothie

Preparation time: 5 minutes

Servings: 2

Ingredients:

ice cubes

1/3 cucumber, cut into 2.5 cm chunks 1 cup of orange juice

1-2 tablespoons fresh ginger, minced 1 cup of coconut yogurt

1 handful fresh baby spinach 7 oz frozen mango chunks

Directions:

1.   Put the ingredients in a food processor.

2.   Blitz until smooth and combined.

3.   Pour into chilled glasses and serve. Enjoy!

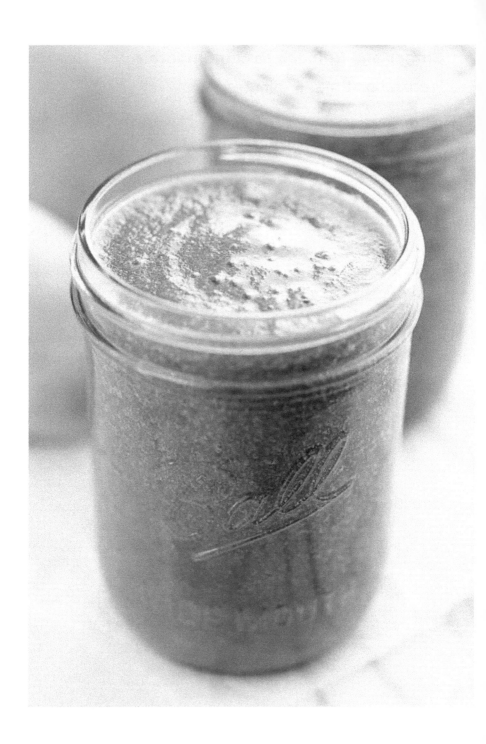

Mint Chocolate Green Protein Smoothie

Preparation Time: 5 minutes

Cooking Time: 10 minutes

Servings: 1 serving

Ingredients:

1 scoop chocolate powder 1 tablespoon flaxseed

1 banana

1 mint leaf

3/4 cup almond milk

3 tablespoons dark chocolate (chopped)

Directions:

1.   Blend the ingredients except chocolate.

2.   Garnish dark chocolate when ready.

Nutrition:

Calories: 300 Fat: 19.1g Carbohydrates: 21.5g Protein: 27.9g

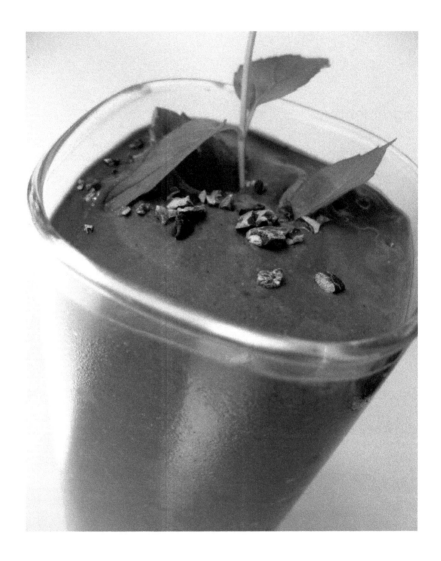

Strawberry Smoothie Bowl

Total time: 30 minutes

Ingredients:

Smoothie bowl:

1 banana frozen

1½ cups frozen strawberries

½ cup coconut milk

Toppings:

Fresh strawberries sliced Fresh bananas sliced Chia seeds

Directions:

1.   In a blender jug, puree all the ingredients for the smooth bowl.

2.   Pour the smoothie into the serving bowl.

3.   Add strawberries, banana, and chia seeds on top.

4.   Chill well, then serve.

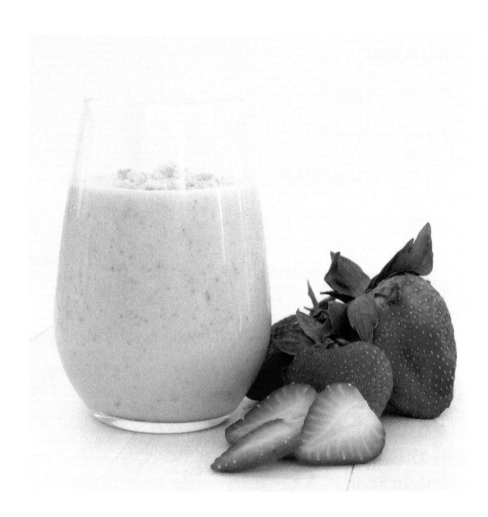

Max Power Smoothie

Preparation Time: 5 minutes

Cooking Time: 0 minute

Servings: 3 to 4 cups

Ingredients:

1 banana

¼ cup rolled oats, or 1 scoop plant Protein: powder 1 tablespoon flaxseed, or chia seeds

1 cup raspberries or other berries

1 cup chopped mango (frozen or fresh)

½ cup non-dairy milk (optional) 1 cup water

Directions:

1.   Purée everything in a blender until smooth, adding more water (or non-dairy milk) if needed.

2.   Add none, some, or all of the bonus boosters, as desired. Purée until blended.

Nutrition:Calories: 550 Fat: 9g Carbs: 116g Fiber: 29g Protein: 13g

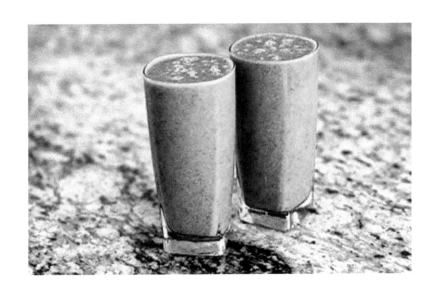

Chocolate Peanutbutter Smoothie

Preparation Time: 5 minutes

Cooking Time: 0 minute

Servings: 3 to 4 cups

Ingredients:

1 banana

¼ cup rolled oats, or 1 scoop plant Protein: powder 1 tablespoon flaxseed, or chia seeds

1 tablespoon unsweetened cocoa powder

1 tablespoon peanut butter, or almond or sunflower seed butter 1 tablespoon maple syrup (optional)

1 cup alfalfa sprouts or spinach, chopped (optional)

½ cup non-dairy milk (optional) 1 cup water

Directions:

1.   Purée everything in a blender until smooth, adding more water (or non-dairy milk) if needed.

2.   Add bonus boosters, as desired. Purée until blended.

Nutrition:

Calories: 474 Fat: 16g Carbs: 79g Fiber: 18g Protein: 13g

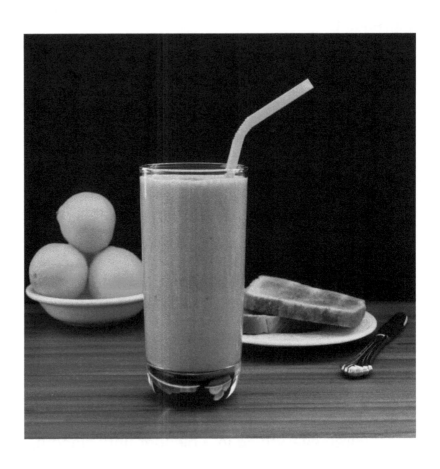

Pink Panther Smoothie

Preparation Time: 5 minutes

Cooking Time: 0 minute

Servings: 3 cups

Ingredients:

1 cup strawberries

1 cup chopped melon (any kind) 1 cup cranberries or raspberries one tablespoon chia seeds

½ cup coconut milk 1 cup water

Directions:

1.   Purée everything in a blender until smooth, adding more water (or coconut milk) if needed.

2.   Add bonus boosters, as desired. Purée until blended.

Nutrition:

Calories: 459 Fat: 30g Carbs: 52g Fiber: 19g Protein: 8g

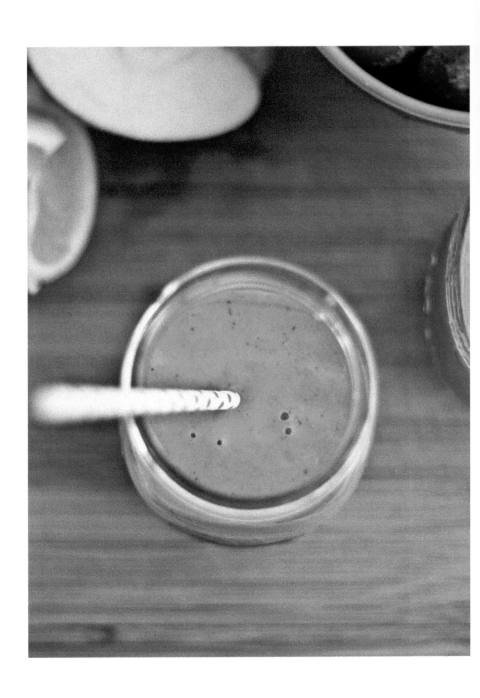

Berry Banana Smoothie Bowl

Cooking time: 10 minutes

Servings: 1

Ingredients

1 cup frozen pineapple

2 tablespoons unsweetened coconut flakes

1/2 cup unsweetened almond milk

1/4 cup blackberries

1 cup baby spinach leaves

10 salted almonds, crushed

2 tablespoons chia seeds

1 banana, sliced

1 cup frozen blueberries

1/2 cup carrots, chopped

Directions:

1. Add all the smoothie ingredients (except coconut flakes, blackberries, and crushed almonds) to a high-speed blender.

2. Blitz to combine until smooth and creamy, then serve.

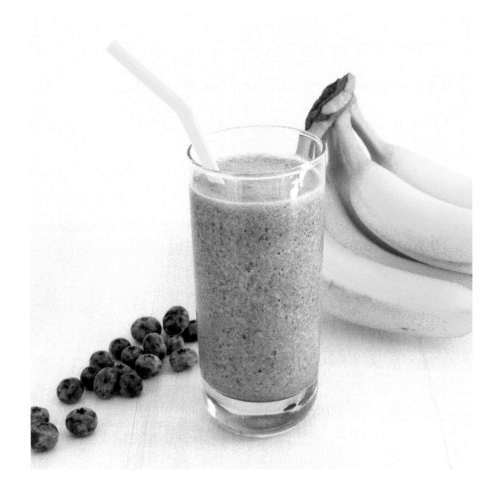

Apple Smoothie

Preparation time: 5 minutes

Cook time: 0 minutes

Serves 2

Ingredients:

1 sweet, crisp apples, cut into 1-inch cubes 2 cups plant-based milk

1 cup ice

1 tablespoon maple syrup

1 tsp cinnamon 1 tsp vanilla extract

Directions:

1. In a blender, combine the apples, milk, ice, maple syrup, cinnamon, and vanilla. Blend until smooth and creamy, then serve.

Per Serving

calories: 198 | fat: 6g | carbs: 32g | protein: 3g | fiber: 8g

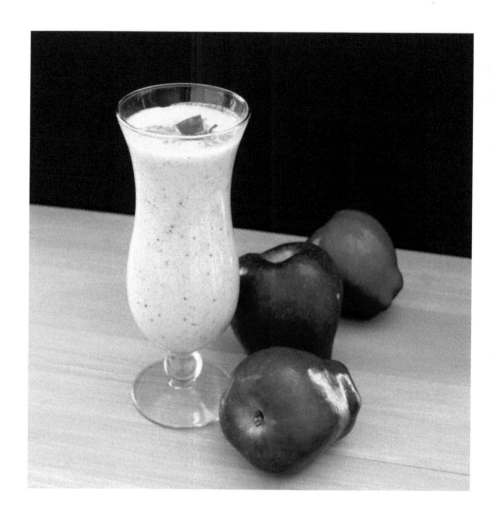

Vitamin C Smoothie Cubes

Preparation time: 5 minutes

Cook time: 0 minutes

Makes 8 smoothies

Ingredients:

1 large papaya

1 mango

2 cups chopped pineapple, fresh or frozen

1 cup raw cauliflower florets, fresh or frozen 2 large navel oranges, peeled and halved

1 orange bell pepper

Directions:

1.   Halve the papaya and mango, remove the pits, and scoop their soft flesh into a high-speed blender.

2.   Add the pineapple, cauliflower, oranges, and bell pepper. Blend until smooth.

3.   Evenly divide the purée between 2 (16-compartment) ice cube trays and place on a level surface in your freezer. Freeze for at least 8 hours.

4.   The cubes can be left in the ice cube trays until use or transferred to a freezer bag. The frozen cubes are good for about 3 weeks in a standard freezer or up to 6 months in a chest freezer.

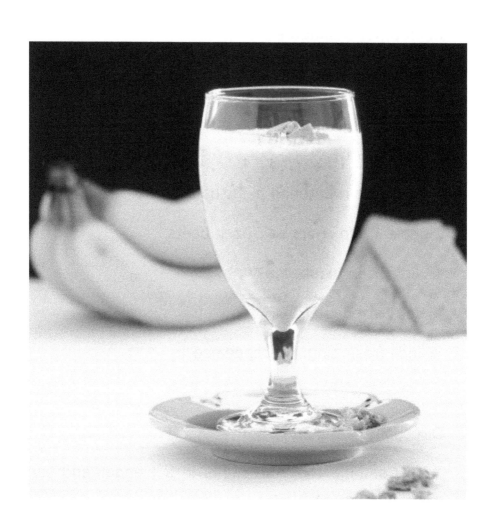

Beet Fruit Smoothie

Preparation time: 5 minutes

Cook time: 0 minutes

Serves 1

Ingredients:

1½ cups unsweetened plant-based milk

1 apple 1 cup chopped frozen beets

1 cup frozen blueberries

½ cup frozen cherries

¼-inch fresh ginger root, peeled

Directions:

1.   Combine the ingredients in a blender and serve. Store in a resealable jar.

Nutrition Per Serving:

calories: 324 | fat: 5g | carbs: 70g | protein: 5g | fiber: 15g

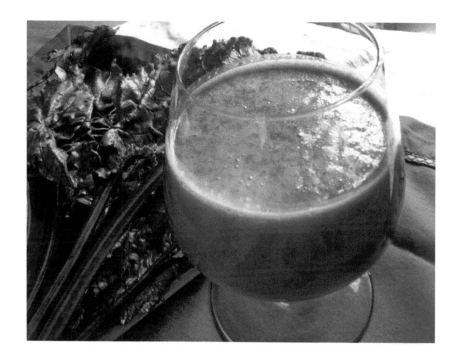

Banana and Mango Smoothie Bowls

Preparation time: 5 minutes

Cook time: 0 minutes

Serves 2

Ingredients:

2 bananas 1 cup mango chunks

1 (20-ounce / 567-g) can pineapple chunks, drained 1 (14-ounce / 397-g) can full-fat coconut milk

1 teaspoon vanilla extract Water, for thinning (optional) Hemp seeds, for garnish Cashew butter, for garnish

Chia seeds, for garnish (optional) Starfruit slices, for garnish (optional)

Fresh pitted cherries for garnish (optional)

Directions:

1. Blend the bananas, mango, pineapple, coconut milk, and vanilla until smooth. This smoothie will be thick and may require several starts and stops to scrape the sides down.

2.   Serve in a bowl topped with hemp seeds, cashew butter, chia seeds, starfruit, and cherries (if using). Enjoy as a refreshing drink instead of adding water.

Nutrition Per Serving (1 smoothie):

calories: 678 | fat: 38g | carbs: 89g | protein: 5g | fiber: 8g

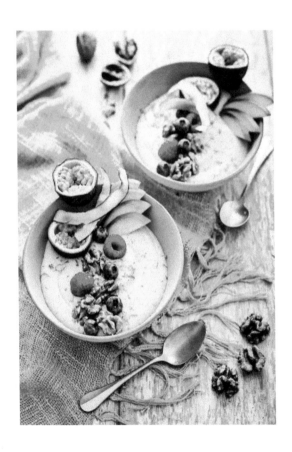

Power Green Smoothie

Preparation time: 5 minutes

Cook time: 0 minutes

Serves 1

Ingredients:

3 cups fresh spinach

1½ cups frozen pineapple

1 cup unsweetened plant-based milk 1 cup fresh kale

1 Granny Smith apple, peeled, cored, and chopped

½ small avocado pitted and peeled

½ teaspoon spirulina

1 tablespoon hemp seeds

Directions:

1.   Combine the ingredients in a blender and serve. Store in a resealable jar.

Nutrition Per Serving:

calories: 431 | fat: 16g | carbs: 70g | protein: 13g | fiber: 17g

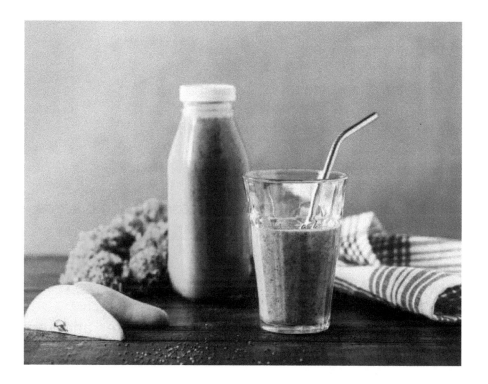

Pineapple Coconut Smoothie

Preparation time: 5 minutes

Cook time: 0 minutes

Serves 1

Ingredients:

2 cups frozen pineapple 1 banana

1¼ cups unsweetened coconut milk

¼ cup frozen coconut pieces

½ teaspoon ground flaxseed 1 teaspoon hemp seeds

Directions:

1. Combine the ingredients in a blender and ser
   Store in a resealable jar.

Nutrition Per Serving

calories: 396 | fat: 14g | carbs: 71g | protein: 6g | fib
11g

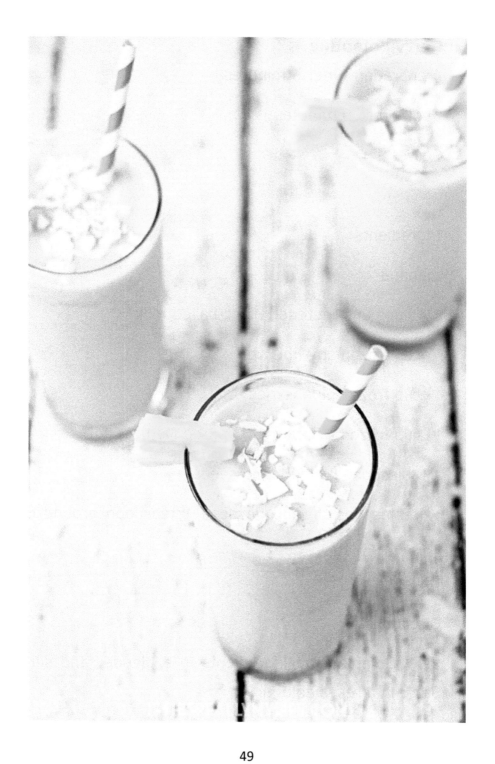

Berry Smoothie

Preparation time: 5 minutes

Cook time: 0 minutes

Serves 1

Ingredients:

 banana

1¼ cups unsweetened plant-based milk

½ cup frozen strawberries

½ cup frozen blueberries

½ cup frozen raspberries 3 pitted Medjool dates

1 tablespoon hulled hemp seeds

½ tablespoon ground flaxseed 1 teaspoon ground chia seeds

Directions:

1.   Combine the ingredients in a blender and serve. Store in a resealable jar.

Nutrition Per Serving:

calories: 538 | fat: 11g | carbs: 111g | protein: 10g |
fiber: 21g

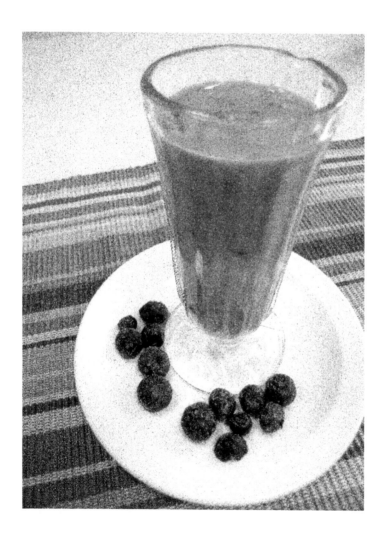

Pumpkin Smoothie

Preparation Time: 5 minutes

Cooking Time: 0 minutes

Servings: 5

Ingredients:

½ cup pumpkin purée

4 Medjool dates 1 cup almond milk

¼ teaspoon vanilla extract

¼ teaspoon ground cinnamon

½ cup ice

Pinch ground nutmeg

Directions:

1.   Combine the ingredients in a blender.

2.   Serve immediately.

Nutrition:

calories: 417 fat: 3.0g carbs: 94.9g fiber: 10.4g protein: 11.4g

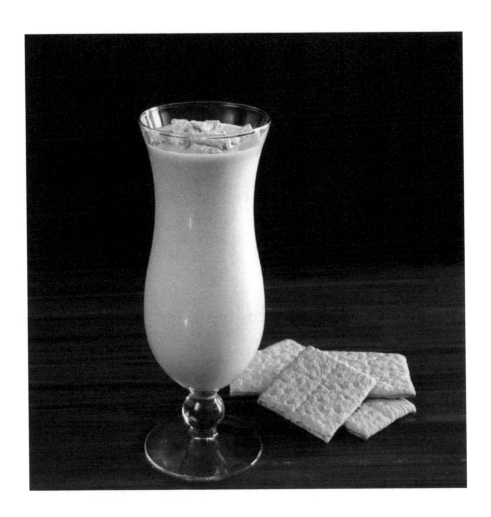

Super Smoothie

Preparation Time: 5 minutes

Cooking Time: 0 minutes

Servings: 4

Ingredients:

1 banana, peeled

1 cup chopped mango 1 cup raspberries

¼ cup rolled oats 1 carrot, peeled

1 cup chopped fresh kale

2 tablespoons chopped fresh parsley 1 tablespo
flaxseeds

1 tablespoon grated fresh ginger

½ cup unsweetened soy milk

1 cup water

Directions:

1.   Put together the ingredients in a food processo
then blitz until glossy and smooth.

2. Serve and enjoy!

Nutrition: calories: 550 fat: 39.0g carbs: 31.0g fiber: 15.0g protein: 13.0g

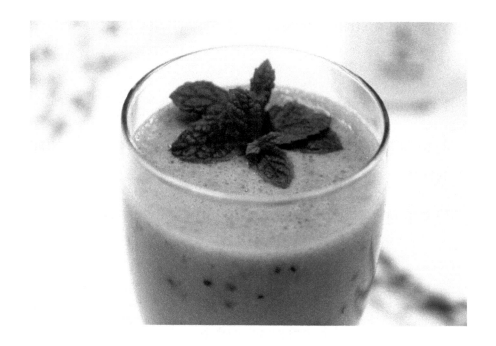

Kiwi and Strawberry Smoothie

Preparation Time: 5 minutes

Cooking Time: 0 minutes

Servings: 3

Ingredients:

1 kiwi, peeled

5 medium strawberries

½ frozen banana

1 cup almond milk 2 tbsp hemp seeds

2 tablespoons peanut butter 1 to 2 teaspoons maple syrup

½ cup spinach leaves Handful broccoli sprouts

Directions:

1.   In a food processor, put together the ingredients, then blitz until creamy and smooth.

2.   Serve and enjoy!

Nutrition: calories: 562 fat: 28.6g carbs: 63.6g fiber: 15.1g protein: 23.3g

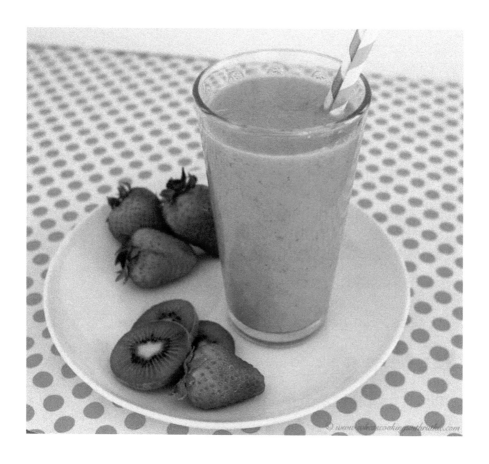

Banana and Chai Chia Smoothie

Preparation Time: 5 minutes

Cooking Time: 0 minutes

Servings: 3

Ingredients:

1 banana

1 cup alfalfa sprouts

1 tablespoon chia seeds

½ cup unsweetened coconut milk 1 to 2 soft Medjool dates, pitted

¼ teaspoon ground cinnamon

1 tablespoon grated fresh ginger 1 cup water

Pinch ground cardamom

Directions:

1. Put together the ingredients in a blender, then process until the mixture is smooth and creamy. Add water or coconut milk if necessary.

2. Serve immediately.

Nutrition: calories: 477 fat: 41.0g carbs: 31.0g fiber: 14.0g protein: 8.0g

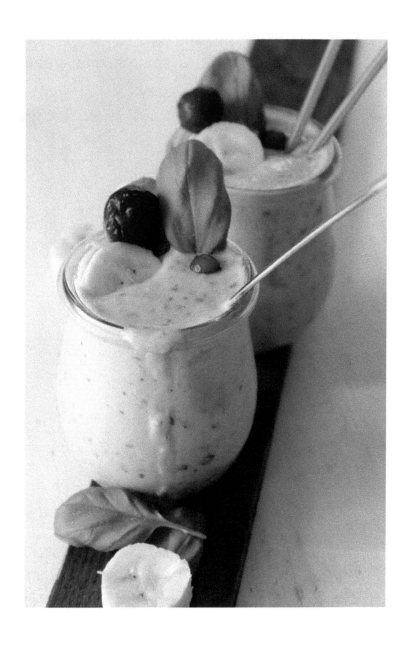

Golden Milk

Preparation Time: 5 minutes

Cooking Time: 0 minutes

Servings: 4

Ingredients:

¼ teaspoon ground cinnamon

½ teaspoon ground turmeric

½ tsp ginger 1 tsp maple syrup

1 cup unsweetened coconut milk Ground black pepper, to taste

2 tablespoon water

Directions:

1.   Combine all the ingredients in a saucepan. Stir to mix well.

2.   Heat over medium heat for 5 minutes. Keep stirring during the heating.

3.   Pour in a blender. Pulse until creamy and smooth. Serve immediately.

Nutrition:

calories: 577 fat: 57.3g carbs: 19.7g fiber: 6.1g Protein: 5.7g

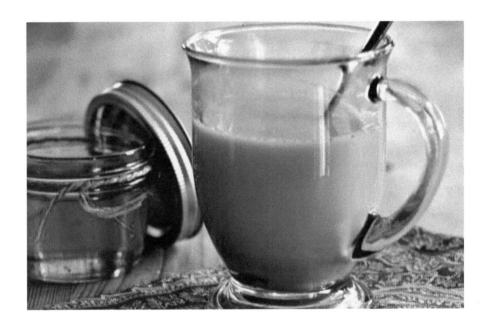

Mango Agua Fresca

Preparation Time: 5 minutes

Cooking Time: 0 minutes

Servings: 2

Ingredients:

2 fresh mangoes, diced 1½ cups water

1   teaspoon fresh lime juice Maple syrup, to taste

2   cups ice

2 slices fresh lime, for garnish 2 fresh mint sprigs, for garnish

Directions:

1.   Put the mangoes, lime juice, maple syrup, and water in a blender. Process until creamy and smooth.

2.   Divide the beverage into two glasses, then garnish each glass with ice, lime slice, and mint sprig before serving.

Nutrition: calories: 230 fat: 1.3g carbs: 57.7g fiber: 5.4g protein: 2.8g

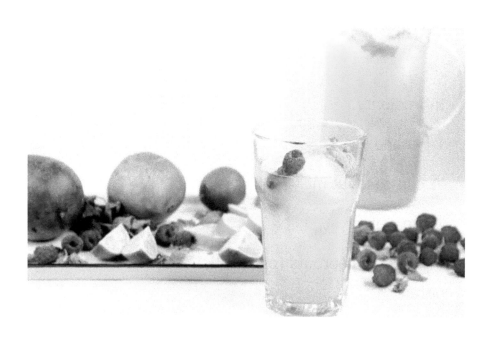

Chai Chia Smoothie

Preparation Time: 5 minutes

Cooking Time: 0 minute

Servings: 3 cups

Ingredients:

1 banana

½ cup coconut milk

1 cup water

1 cup alfalfa sprouts (optional) 1 to 2 soft Medjool dates, pitted

1 tbsp chia seeds

¼ teaspoon ground cinnamon Pinch ground cardamom

1 tablespoon grated fresh ginger or ¼ teaspoon ground ginger

Directions:

1.   Purée everything in a blender until smooth, adding more water (or coconut milk) if needed.

Nutrition:

Calories: 477 Fat: 29g Carbs: 57g Fiber: 14g Protein: 8g

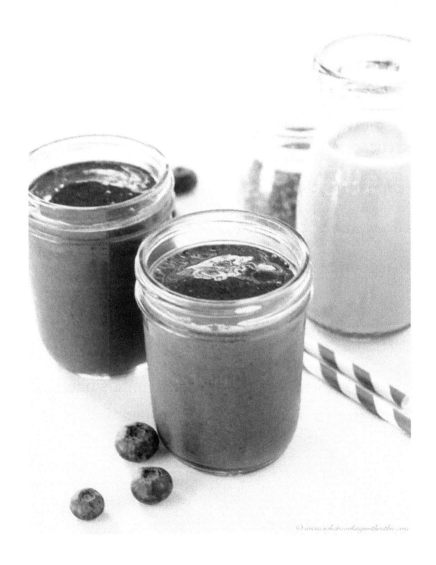

Trope-Kale Breeze

Preparation Time: 5 minutes

Cooking Time: 0 minute

Servings: 3 to 4 cups

Ingredients:

1 cup chopped pineapple (frozen or fresh) 1 cup chopped mango (frozen or fresh)

½ to 1 cup chopped kale

½ avocado

½ cup coconut milk

1 cup water or coconut water

1 teaspoon matcha green tea powder (optional)

Directions:

1.   Purée everything in a blender until smooth, adding more water (or coconut milk) if needed.

Nutrition:

Calories: 566 Fat: 36g Carbs: 66g Fiber: 12g Protein: 8g

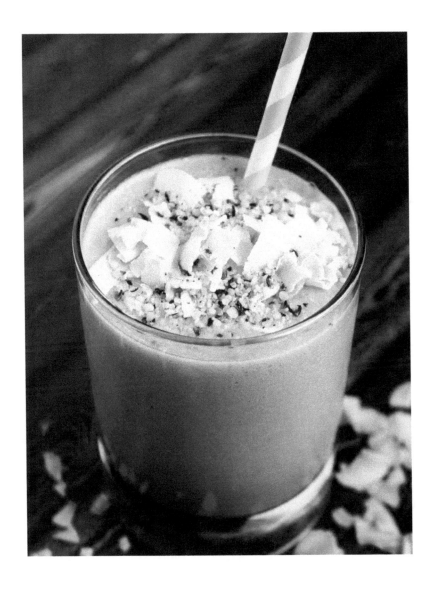

Hydration Station

Preparation Time: 5 minutes

Cooking Time: 0 minute

Servings: 3 to 4 cups

Ingredients:

1 banana

1 orange, peeled and sectioned, or 1 cup pure orange juice 1 cup strawberries (frozen or fresh)

1 cup chopped cucumber

½ cup coconut water 1 cup water

½ cup ice

Directions:

1. Purée everything in a blender until smooth, adding more water if needed.

Add bonus boosters, as desired. Purée until blended.

Nutrition:

Calories: 320 Fat: 3g Carbs: 76g Fiber: 13g Protein: 6g

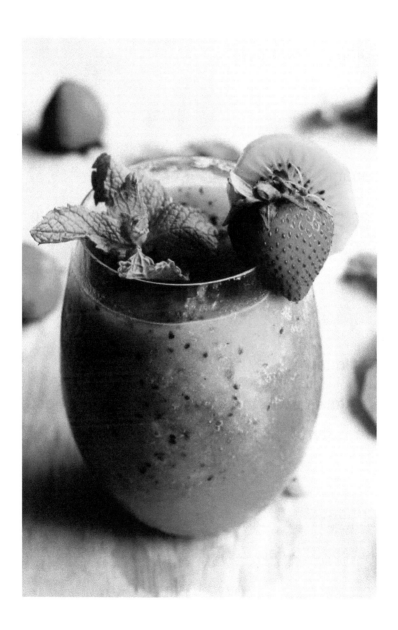

Mango Madness

Preparation Time: 5 minutes

Cooking Time: 0 minute

Servings: 3 to 4 cups

Ingredients:

1 banana

1 cup chopped mango (frozen or fresh) 1 cup chopped peach (frozen or fresh) 1 cup strawberries

1 carrot 1 cup water

Directions:

1.   Purée everything in a blender until smooth, adding more water if needed.

Nutrition:

Calories: 376 Fat: 2g Carbs: 95g Fiber: 14g Protein: 5g

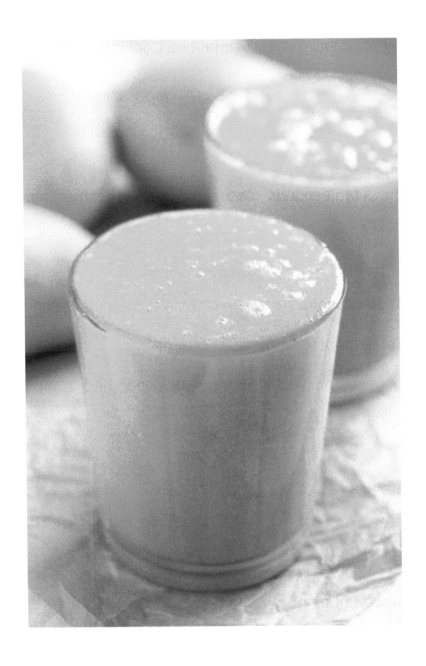

Brownie Batter Orange Chia Shake

Preparation Time: 5 minutes Cooking Time: 0 minute
Servings: 2

Ingredients:

2 tablespoons cocoa powder 3 tablespoons chia seeds

¼ teaspoon salt

4 tablespoons chocolate chips 4 teaspoons coconut sugar

½ teaspoon orange zest

½ teaspoon vanilla extract, unsweetened 2 cup almond milk

Directions:

1. Blend the ingredients for 2 to 3 minutes at high speed until smooth.

2. Pour the smoothie into two glasses and then serve.

Nutrition: Calories: 290 Fat: 11g Protein: 20g Sugar: 9g

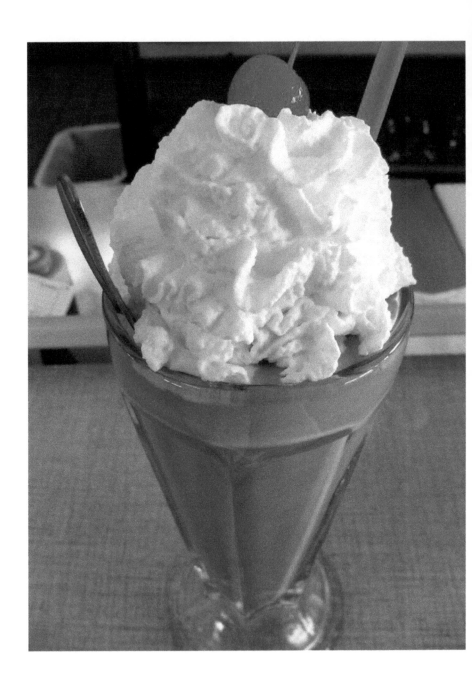

Bracing Coffee Smoothie

Preparation Time: 5 minutes

Cooking Time: 5 minutes

Servings: 1

Ingredients:

1 banana, sliced and frozen

½ cup strong brewed coffee

½ cup milk

¼ cup rolled oats 1 tsp nut butter

Directions:

1.   Mix all the ingredients until smooth.

2.   Enjoy your morning drink!

Nutrition:

Calories 414 Fat 20.6 g Carbohydrates 5.6 g Sugar 1.3 g Protein 48.8 g Cholesterol 58 mg

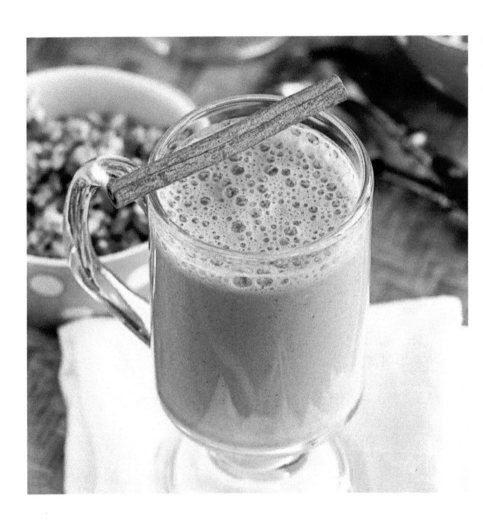

Vitamin Green Smoothie

Preparation Time: 5 minutes

Cooking Time: 5 minutes

Servings: 2

Ingredients:

1 cup milk or juice

1 cup spinach or kale

½ cup plain yogurt 1 kiwi

1 Tbsp chia or flax 1 tsp vanilla

Directions:

1.   Mix the milk or juice and greens until smooth. Add the remaining ingredients and continue blending until smooth again.

2.   Enjoy your delicious drink!

Nutrition:

Calories 397 Fat 36.4 g Carbohydrates 4 g Sugar 1 g Protein 14.7 g Cholesterol 4 mg

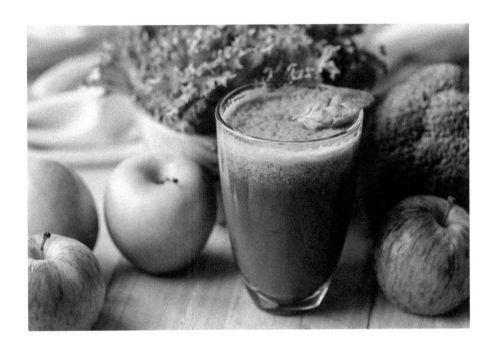

Strawberry Grapefruit Smoothie

Preparation Time: 5 minutes

Cooking Time: 5 minutes

Servings: 2

Ingredients:

1 banana

½ cup strawberries, frozen 1 grapefruit

¼ cup milk

¼ cup plain yogurt 2 Tbsp honey

½ tsp ginger, chopped

Directions:

1.   Using a mixer, blend all the ingredients.

2.   When smooth, top your drink with a slice of grapefruit and enjoy it!

Nutrition:

Calories 233 Fat 7.9 g Carbohydrates 3.2 g Sugar 0.1 g Protein 35.6 g Cholesterol 32 m

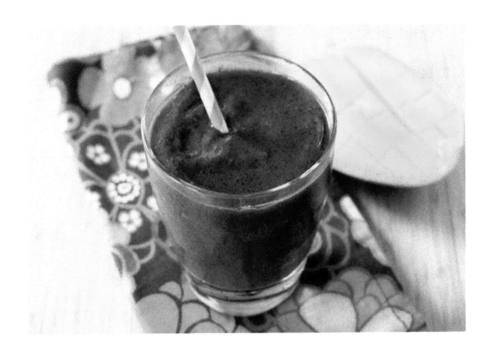

Inspirational Orange Smoothie

Preparation Time: 5 minutes

Cooking Time: 5 minutes

Servings: 1

Ingredients:

4 mandarin oranges, peeled 1 banana, sliced and frozen

½ cup non-fat yogurt

1 cup fresh coconut water 1 tsp pure vanilla extract 5 ice cubes

Directions:

1.   Using a mixer, whisk all the ingredients.

2.   Enjoy your drink!

Nutrition:

Calories 256 Fat 13.3 g Carbohydrates 0 g Sugar 0 g Protein 34.5 g Cholesterol 78 mg

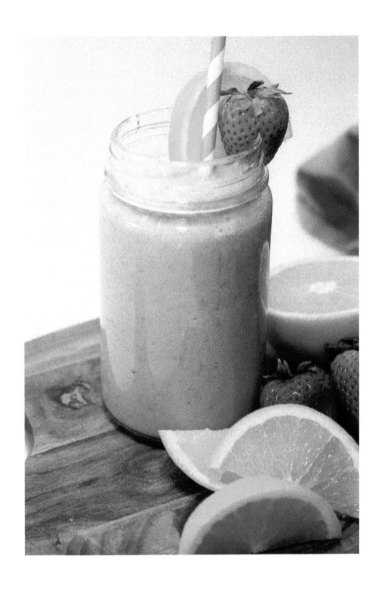

Mint Banana Smoothie

Preparation time: 5 minutes

Cook time: 0 minutes

Serves 2

Ingredients:

2 cups plant-based milk 2 frozen bananas, halved

1 tablespoon fresh mint leaves or ¼ teaspoon peppermint extract 1 teaspoon vanilla extract

Directions:

1.   Combine the ingredients in a blender and serve. Store in a resealable jar.

Nutrition Per Serving:

calories: 152 | fat: 4g | carbs: 30g | protein: 2g | fiber: 4g

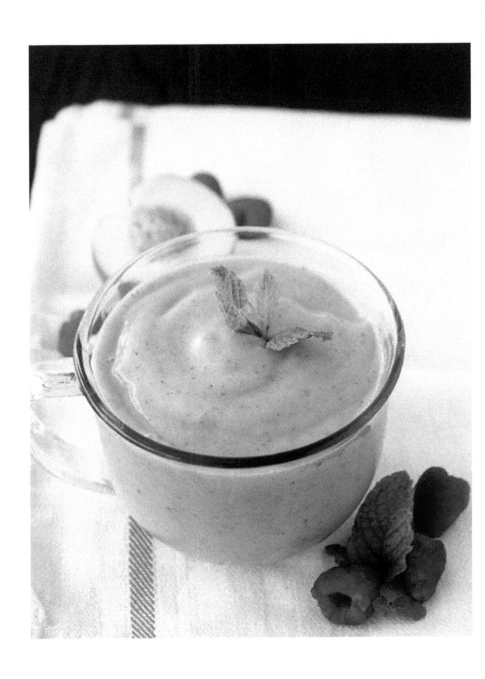

Sunshine Orange Smoothie

Preparation Time: 5 minutes

Cooking Time: 0 minutes

Servings: 4

Ingredients:

2 medium oranges, zested, juiced 4 frozen bananas

4 tablespoons goji berries

½ cup hemp seeds

1 teaspoon grated ginger

1 cup almond milk, unsweetened

½ cup of ice cubes

Directions:

1.   Blender and then pulse for 1 to 2 minutes until blended, scraping the container's sides frequently.

2.   Distribute the smoothie among glasses and then serve.

Nutrition:

Calories: 131 Fat: 2.3g Carbs: 26.7g Sugars: 11g Protein: 2.6g

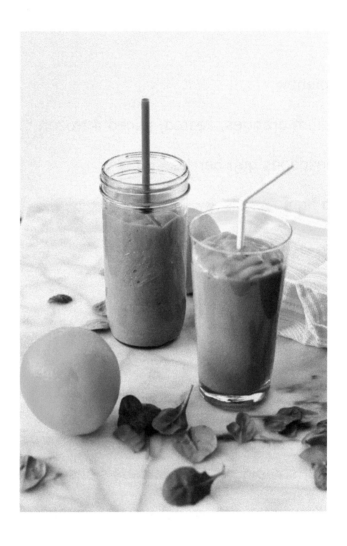

Chocolate and Hazelnut Smoothie

Preparation Time: 5 minutes

Cooking Time: 0 minutes

Servings: 4

Ingredients:

1 frozen banana

1 cup hazelnuts, unsalted, roasted 8 teaspoons maple syrup

4 tablespoons cocoa powder, unsweetened 1/2 teaspoon hazelnut extract, unsweetened 2 cups almond milk, unsweetened

1 cup of ice cubes

Directions:

1.   Blender and then pulse for 1 to 2 minutes until blended, scraping the container's sides frequently.

2.   Distribute the smoothie among glasses and then serve.

Nutrition:

Calories: 198 Fat: 12g Carbs: 21g Sugars: 12g Protein: 5g

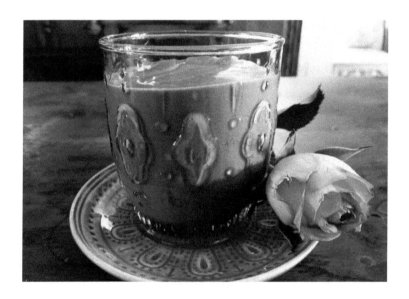

Blueberry Oatmeal Smoothie

Preparation Time: 5 minutes

Cooking Time: 0 minutes

Servings: 4

Ingredients:

2 cups frozen blueberries 1 cup old-fashioned oats 2 teaspoons cinnamon

2 tablespoons maple syrup 1 cup spinach

2 cup almond milk, unsweetened 8 ice cubes

Directions:

1.   Blender and then pulse for 1 to 2 minutes until blended, scraping the container's sides frequently.

2.   Distribute the smoothie among glasses and then serve.

Nutrition:

Calories: 194 Fat: 5g Carbs: 34g Sugars: 15g Protein: 5g

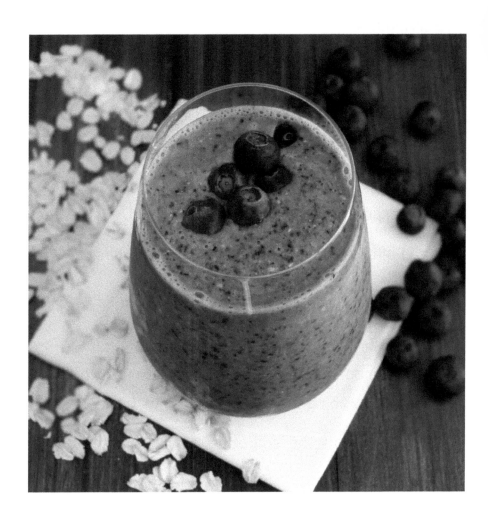

Pear and Apple Smoothie

Preparation time: 2 minutes

Cook time: 4 minutes

Makes 3 cups

Ingredients:

2 (1-pound / 454-g) large firm but ripe pears, peeled, quartered, and cored 2 (1-pound / 454-g) large apples, peeled, quartered, and cored

¼ cup apple juice

Directions:

1.	Put the ingredients in the pot. Cook for 4 minutes at low pressure.

2.	Open the pot.

3.	Use a hand mixer to break the pears and apples to make the smoothie.

4.	Serve immediately.

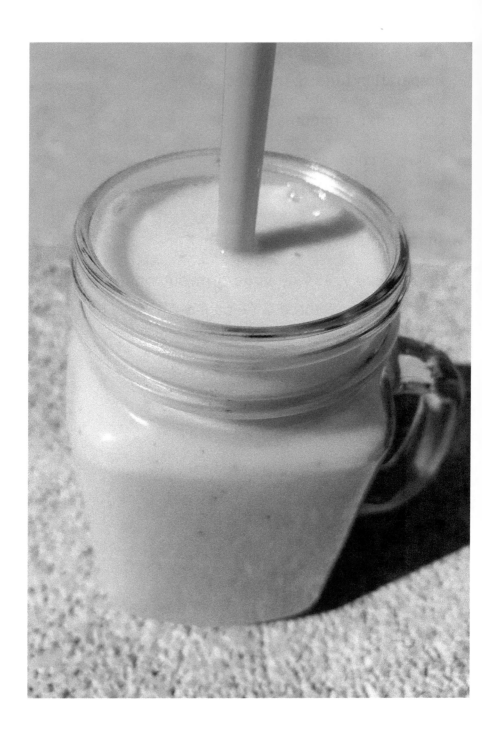

Kale Smoothie

Preparation Time: 5 minutes

Cooking Time: 0 minutes

Servings: 2

Ingredients:

2 cups chopped kale leaves 1 banana, peeled

1 cup frozen strawberries

1 cup unsweetened almond milk

4 Medjool dates, pitted and chopped

Directions:

1.   Put the ingredients in a food processor, then blitz until glossy and smooth.

2.   Serve immediately.

Nutrition: calories: 663 fat: 10.0g carbs: 142.5g fiber: 19.0g protein: 17.4g

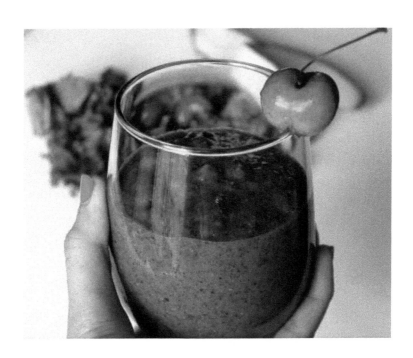

Hot Tropical Smoothie

Preparation Time: 5 minutes

Cooking Time: 0 minutes

Servings: 4

Ingredients:

1 cup frozen mango chunks

1 cup frozen pineapple chunks

1 small tangerine, peeled and pitted 2 cups spinach leaves

1 cup coconut water

¼ teaspoon cayenne pepper, optional

Directions:

1.   Blitz the ingredients until the mixture is smooth and combine well.

2.   Serve and enjoy!

Nutrition:

calories: 283 fat: 1.9g carbs: 67.9g fiber: 10.4g protein: 6.4g

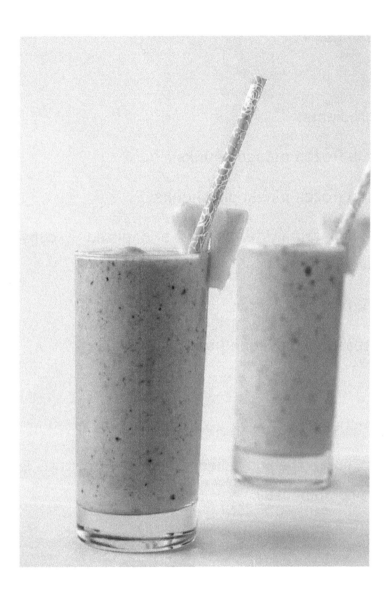

Cranberry and Banana Smoothie

Preparation Time: 5 minutes

Cooking Time: 0 minutes

Servings: 4

Ingredients:

1 cup frozen cranberries 1 large banana, peeled

4 Medjool dates, pitted and chopped 1½ cups unsweetened almond milk

Directions:

1.   Mix the ingredients until glossy.

2.   Serve and enjoy!

Nutrition:

calories: 616 fat: 8.0g carbs: 132.8g fiber: 14.6g protein: 15.7g

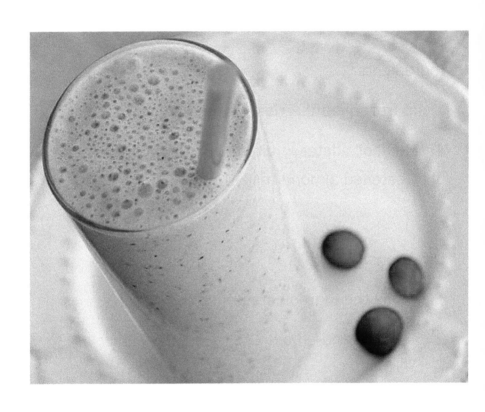

Cookie Dough Smoothie

Preparation Time: 5 minutes

Cooking Time: 0 minutes

Servings: 4

Ingredients:

4 frozen banana

8 tablespoons hemp seeds

8 tablespoons chocolate chips, vegan 4 scoops of salted caramel Protein:

2 teaspoons cinnamon

8 teaspoons honey

8 tablespoons peanut butter powder 4 cups almond milk, unsweetened 4 cups of ice cubes

Directions:

1.   Blender and then pulse for 1 to 2 minutes until blended, scraping the container's sides frequently.

2.   Distribute the smoothie among glasses and then serve.

Nutrition:

Calories: 442 Fat: 19.5g Carbs: 41.3g Sugars: 22.2g Protein: 31.2g

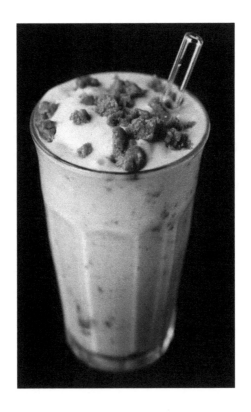

Coffee Smoothie

Preparation Time: 5 minutes

Cooking Time: 0 minutes

Servings: 4

Ingredients:

4 cups baby spinach

4 tablespoons hemp hearts 12 Medjool dates, pitted

4 tablespoons cashew butter 2 cups brewed coffee, chilled 6 cups of ice cubes

Directions:

1.   Let the pitted dates soak for 15 minutes.

2.   Drain the dates, put togethe with the remaining ingredients, and then pulse for 1 to 2 minutes until blended, scraping the sides of the container frequently.

3.   Distribute the smoothie among glasses and then serve.

Nutrition:

Calories: 391 Fat: 15g Carbs: 60g Sugars: 47g Protein: 10g

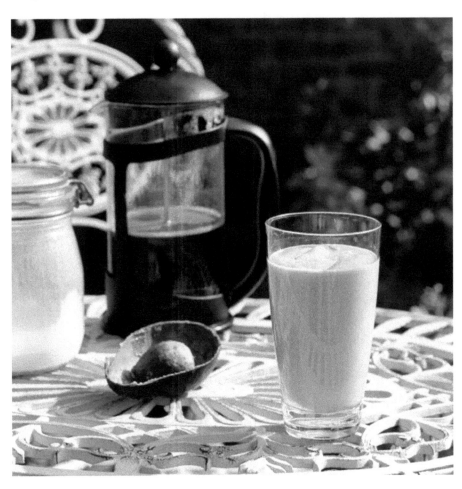

Almond Milk Banana Smoothie

Cook time: 5 minutes

Servings: 1

Ingredients

1 banana, frozen

¾ cup almond milk

3 tbsp peanutbutter 2 tbsp cacao powder

For topping:

½ banana, sliced Chocolate granola

Instructions

1.   Blend bananas, almond milk, peanut butter, and cacao powder in a blender until smooth.

2.   Serve in a bowl and enjoy!

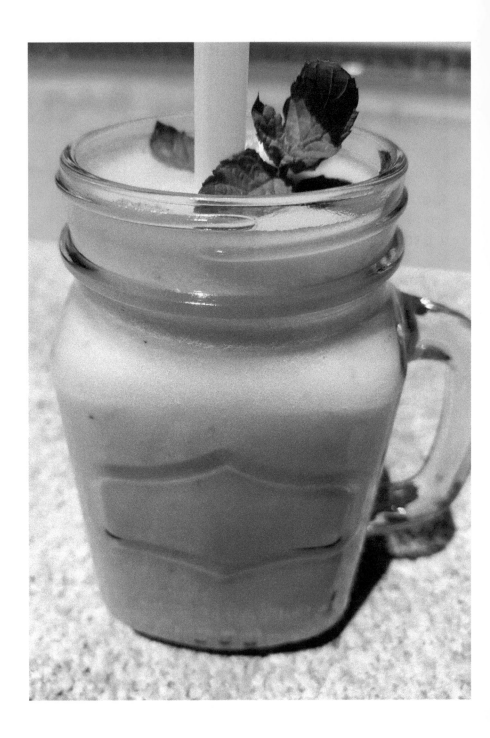

Chocolate Black Bean Smoothie

Cook Time: 2 minutes

Servings: 1

Ingredients:

1 cup cauliflower, frozen 1 banana, frozen

1/2 cup black beans 1 cup almond milk 1/2 Medjool dates

1 tablespoon cocoa powder 1 tablespoon hemp seeds

1 teaspoon ground cinnamon

Instructions:

1.   Blend all the ingredients until smooth.

2.   Transfer to a glass cup and serve.

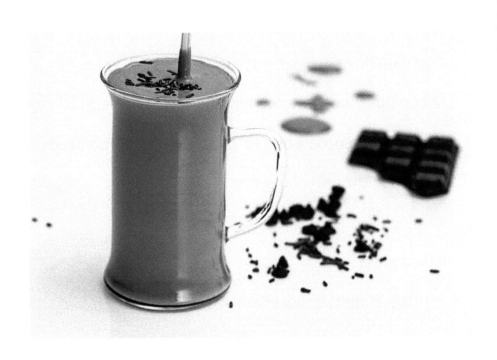

Youthful Green Smoothie

Preparation time: 5 minutes

Servings: 4

Ingredients

1/2 cucumber

1 teaspoon fresh ginger, grated

2 handfuls kale or power greens mix ice

2 oz baby spinach 1 banana

2 cups apple juice 1/2 lemon, squeezed

Instructions:

1.   Put the ingredients in a food processor.

2.   Blitz until smooth and combined.

3.   Pour into chilled glasses and serve. Enjoy!

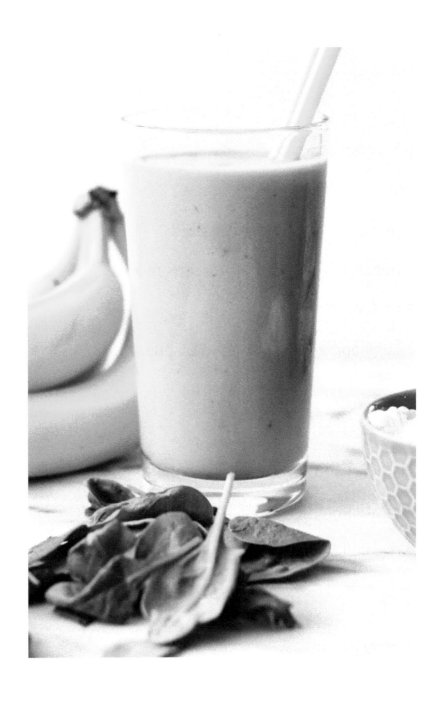

Lightning Source UK Ltd.
Milton Keynes UK
UKHW020647300421
382892UK00001B/53